The Qi-Life:
Live A Better Life Pain Free Naturally

Other titles by Dr. Michele Arnold-Pirtle:

Ancient Healing for Modern People: Food, Herbs & Essential Oils to De tox, Cleanse & Rejuvenate the Body, Mind & Soul

Medicine Mom's Essential Oil Recipes & Everything Holistic: Natura Remedies for Common Ailments

A free eBook download with subscription to Acupuncture Center Inc., *The Top 6 Alternatives to Rx Pain Killers: Live A Better Life Pain Free Naturally.*

Essential Renewal: A Chinese Medicine 30-Day Cleanse Using Essentia Oils, Natural Supplements, and Whole Foods to Rejuvenate Your Gut and Your Life! For sale directly by author, while supplies last. A Gut cleanse and renewal using dietary practices of Chinese Medicine along with doTERRA essential oils and supplements.

The Qi-Life:
Live A Better Life Pain Free Naturally

Dr. Michele Arnold-Pirtle

Total Health Acupuncture Center
2019

Disclaimer

This book has not been evaluated by the FDA. The products and methods recommended are not intended to treat, diagnose, cure, or prevent illness or disease. It is not a substitute for medical advice.

This book has been designed to provide information to help educate the reader regarding the subject matter covered. It is made available with the understanding that the author and publisher is not liable for any misconception or misuse of the information provided. The author and publisher shall have neither liability nor responsibility to any person or entity with respect to any loss, damage or injury cased or alleged to be caused, directly or indirectly by the information contained in this book. The information presented herein is in no way intended as a substitute for medical counseling. Anyone suffering from any disease, illness, or injury should consult a qualified health care professional.

Any mention of Bio-Medical Disease Names, Common Disease Names, or Symptoms does not claim the ability of Chinese herbal formulas, essential oils, whole foods, or supplements to cure, treat, heal or prevent, such conditions. The names are included only for clarification of common support for minor and occasional everyday wellness needs

Copyright © 2019 by Dr. Michele Arnold-Pirtle

First Printing: 2019

ISBN 9781797436517

Total Health Acupuncture Center

15644 Pomerado Rd., Ste. 102

Poway, CA 92064

www.acupuncturecenterinc.com

Credit Artwork Shutterstock.com

Dedication

To my loyal and dear patients for whom I wrote this book.

Thank you. Without your support and patience, I would have never achieved my dream.

Contents

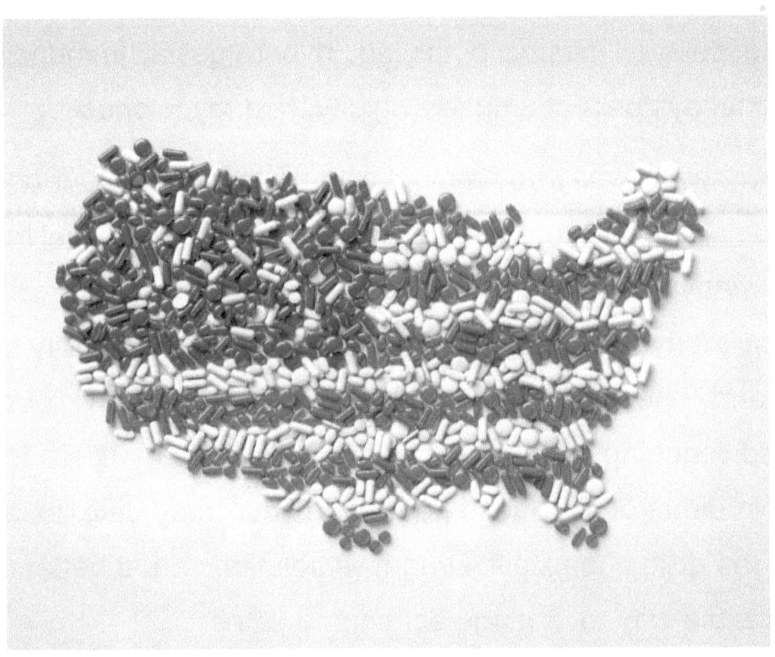

The Rx Drug Crisis

America is in the middle of an opioid crisis! There are more people addicted to pain pills than there are people addicted to heroin and cocaine combined. There are more overdoses from prescription opioid use in the U.S. than any other illegal drug.

While pain pills, steroids, non-steroidal anti-inflammatory (NSAIDS) medications may temporarily relieve your pain, there are many side-effects, contribute to long-term health problems, and they can be highly addictive.

Common side effects of opioid administration include sedation, dizziness, nausea, vomiting, constipation, physical dependence, tolerance, and respiratory depression. Physical dependence and addiction are clinical concerns that may prevent proper prescribing and in turn inadequate pain management. Less common side effects may include delayed gastric emptying, hyperalgesia, immunologic and hormonal dysfunction, muscle rigidity, and myoclonus.

Occasional use may be fine, but with prolonged use our bodies may build up a tolerance requiring higher doses in order to feel the effects. What many people don't realize is that the drugs can cause more pain called hyperalgesia. This reduces your body's ability to tolerate pain, and it becomes more sensitive to it. Thus, a vicious cycle is created requiring the use of more pain relievers. There is also the letdown effect of increased pain while your body detoxes and eliminates the drug chemicals. Drug-free solutions are a better and more responsible way to manage aches and pains.

Holistic and natural ways to improve your health and manage pain that you can do yourself may include using acupressure techniques, stress reduction and meditation, exercise, eating right, losing weight, natural herbal remedies, essential oils, and Hemp Cannabidiol Oil (CBD).

The Qi-Life for Wellness

Daily Guide with Acupressure, Healthy Spleen-Qi Diet, and Enhancing One's Spiritual-Emotional Well-Being.

A life in essential harmony has strong and balanced Qi-energy, vital to health.

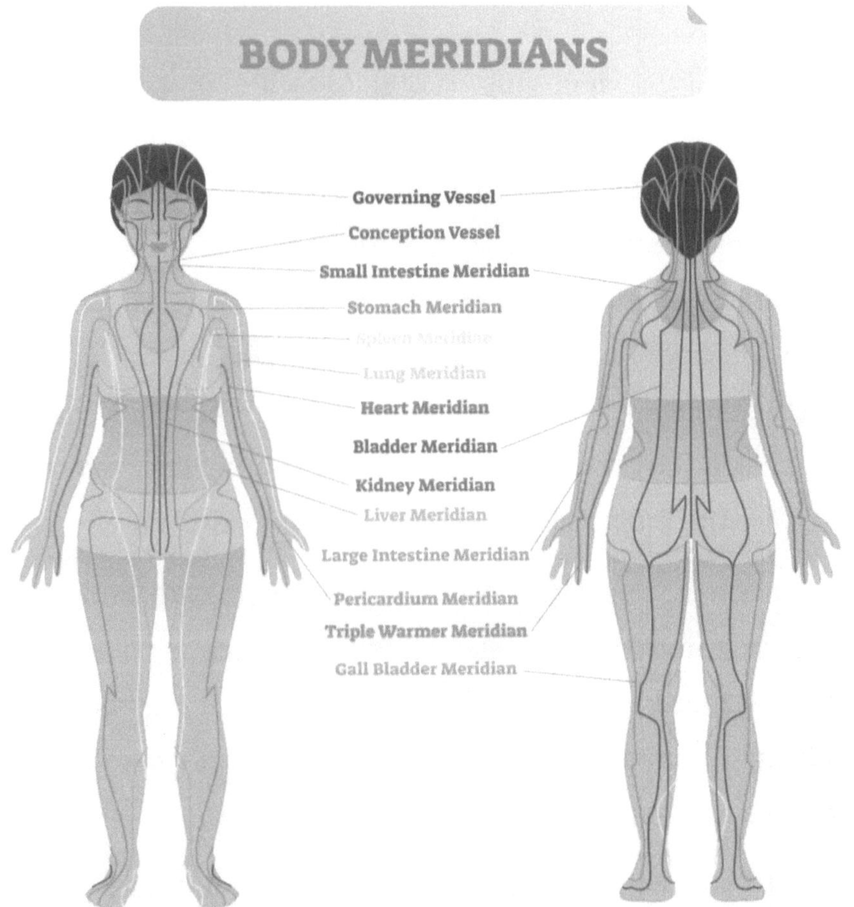

Qi (chee or chi) has many different meanings such as, energy, warmth, breath, air, space, oxygen, movement, or function.

Qi flows in our channel systems and blood vessels. The channels are also called meridians because they look like meridian lines found on a map. They are found superficially on our skin following line like blood vessels and nerves. They reach interiorly connecting to our organs and glands. They are responsible for communication and energy distribution reaching every muscle, organ, gland, tissue, and cell of our body. Thus, they are important for both treatment and diagnosis.

It is important to keep Qi-energy flowing freely that becomes blocked by normal stresses of everyday life. An obstruction to the flow of Qi is like a dam. When Qi becomes backed up in one part of the body, the flow becomes restricted in other parts. This blockage of the flow of Qi can be detrimental to a person's health, cutting off vital nourishment to the body, organs and glands. Physical and emotional trauma, stress, lack of exercise, overexertion, seasonal changes, poor diet, accidents, or excessive activity are among the many things that can influence the quality, quantity and balance of Qi.

Normally, when a blockage or imbalance occurs, the body easily bounces back, returning to a state of health and well-being. However, when this disruption is prolonged or excessive, or if the body is in a weakened state, illness, pain, or disease can set in. According to ancient Chinese Medical theory:

Blockage of the flow of Qi can be detrimental to a person's health and leads to various signs and symptoms or health concerns.

Acupuncturists can provide you with Chinese herbal remedies as well as regular acupuncture treatments that can free the flow of blocked Qi-energy and blood to help keep you feeling healthy and strong. At home methods often recommended by acupuncturists include acupressure, meditation, exercise, massage, essential oils, food therapy for specific complaints, eating a healthy spleen-Qi diet, periodic fasting, or a cleansing and detoxification program.

Acupressure Points and the Meridians

There are fourteen main meridians, with twelve primary paired channels, and two single channels. The primary channels are each named according to the organ it innervates which are, Liver, Gallbladder, Heart, Small Intestine, Pericardium, Triple Warmer, Spleen, Stomach, Lung, Large Intestine, Kidney and Bladder. The two single channels are found along our midline, the conception vessel (Ren) down the front, and the directing or governing vessel (Du) down the back on the spine. Along the channels are spaces, or holes, which are surrounded by a greater density of neural capillary beds, called acupuncture points, or nodes. They act as electrical transmitters along an electrical circuit. Qi coursing through the channels can be manipulated at these stations.

The aim in Chinese Medicine is to restore the proper flow of this Qi energy with proper stimulus via acupuncture, heat, herbs, food, or exercise.

Qi is activated along the channels of the skin when pressed with your thumb as in acupressure, pierced with an acupuncture needle, warmed with the burning of an herb mugwort (moxibustion or moxa), when aromatic oils are applied, color light, micro-current electrical stimulation, or with sound vibration from tuning forks.

Acupressure can be done twice daily with your morning or evening routine. The positive effects are accumulated over time with consistent use. When you are feeling better, and out of pain you can use acupressure once per week to extend results from acupuncture treatments, and to stay balanced.

Use your thumb or index finger to apply gentle yet firm pressure that allows the skin and muscle to move underneath. Move in a clockwise fashion keeping your finger on the point. Hold each point for 30 seconds to one minute or more. Do it until the point becomes heavy, achy, or numb like. Then move on to the next point.

The measurement used is the Chinese inch called cun. It is equal to the width of your thumb.

There are numerous acupuncture points on the body, head, face and ears. The following point selection was chosen because of their easy to find locations, wide array of uses, and effectiveness. Together as a protocol these points open areas of congested Qi-energy and blood, keep circulation moving, benefit the spleen-pancreas, and stomach channels, relax and sooth the liver and gall bladder energies, reduce pain, calm the mind, and lift the mood.

Begin on the left hand, move to left leg, foot, then right foot, leg, then right hand, then center of the body, upper shoulders, and lastly the head.

Large Intestine 4 Union Valley/He Gu. Location: In the middle of the 2nd metacarpal bone on the radial side.   Tip-In the web, between the thumb and first finger, at the highest point when the fingers are together. In the picture below, we are using a tuning fork. Pressure with your finger is effective as well.

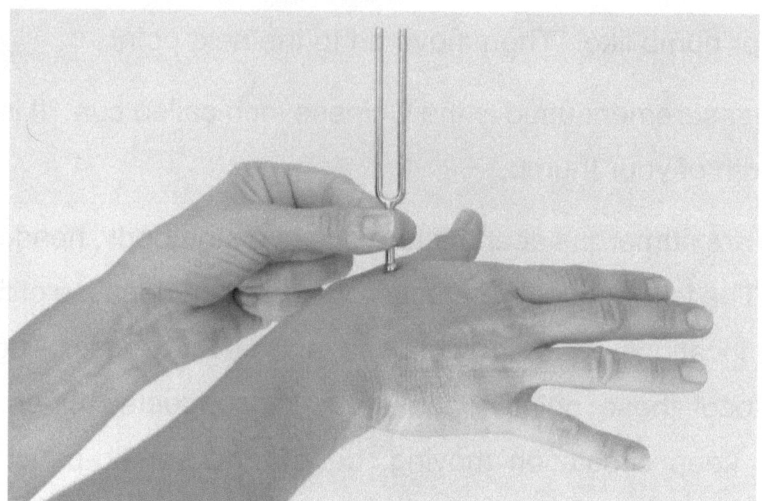

•This point influences the free flow of Qi and blood circulation in the channels, alleviates pain,

•Boosts immunity

•Goes to the head and teeth for headaches and tooth pain, allergies, nasal congestion

•Promotes labor. *Contraindicated during pregnancy.

Pericardium 6 Inner Pass/Nei Guan. Location: 2 finger widths above the wrist crease, in the center, between the tendons of palmaris longus and flexor carpl radlalis. Tip-This might be where your wrist watch goes.

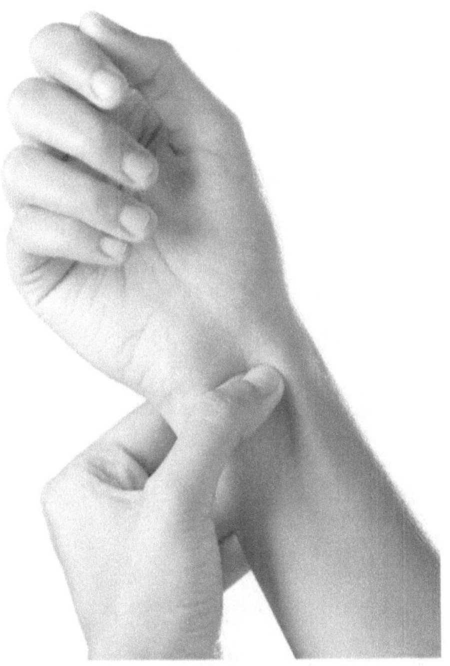

- This point benefits the heart, eases chest constriction, angina, palpitations, asthma.
- Calms the mind, and shen-spirit for insomnia, nervousness, mania, stress, poor memory.
- Supports the digestive system and eases nausea, vomiting, morning sickness, sea sickness, stomach pain.
- Local pain, carpal tunnel syndrome.

Stomach 36 Three Leg Mile/Zusanli. Location: 3 cun below S
36, one finger width lateral from the anterior border of the tibia. Tip
Below the knee, on the outer side, just off the shin bone.

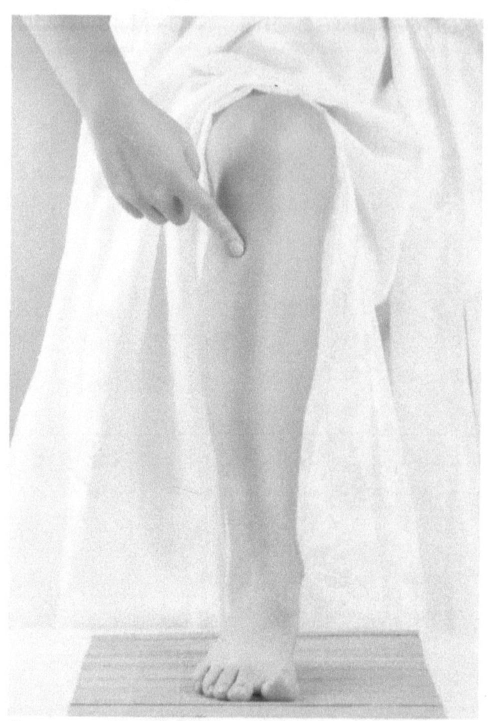

•Boosts immunity, and white blood cell counts.
•Strengthens Qi-energy for general weakness, chronic illness
poor digestion.
•Balances excess or deficient conditions of the spleen-pancreas,
stomach meridians such as constipation, diarrhea, stomach pain
and fullness, rumbling intestines, and GERD.
•Opens the channel to help with breast pain or lower leg pain.
•Supports respiratory functions of lungs for asthma, dyspnea.
•Calms the mind and spirit for depression, nervousness, insom-
nia, PMS

Liver 3 Great Surge/Tai Chong. Location: On the dorsum of the foot in a depression distal to the junctions of the 1st and 2nd metatarsal bones. Tip-On the top of the foot, between the big toe and second toe, in the depression.

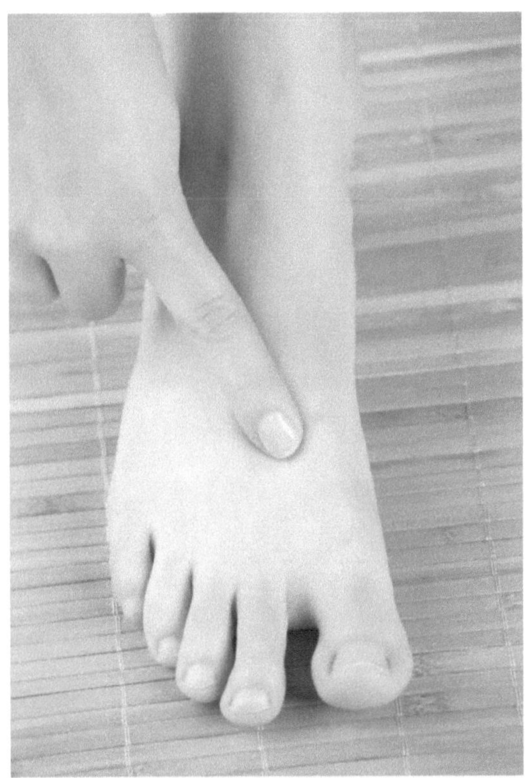

•Powerfully influences the free flow of Qi and blood circulation, alleviates pain especially when used in conjunction with Large Intestine 4.

•Descends rising Yang energies from the head such as headaches, dizziness, canker sores.

•Soothes gynecological issues like PMS, menstrual pain, dysmenorrhea, breast tenderness.

•Genital problems such as hernia, impotence, pain and swelling.

•Congestion in the liver, and subcostal area, chest and flank pain, swellings in the axillary-arm pit area.

•Benefits digestion for nausea, vomiting, constipation, diarrhea.
•Brightens the eyes, soothes red irritated eyes, blurry vision floaters.
•Clams the spirit for anger, irritability, insomnia, anxiety.

Gall Bladder 21 Shoulder Well/Jiang Jing. Location: On the shoulder directly above the nipple at the midpoint of a line connecting GV 14 and the acromion at the highest point of the shoulder. Tip-Highest point on the shoulder, midway between the shoulder joint and the junction of the neck.

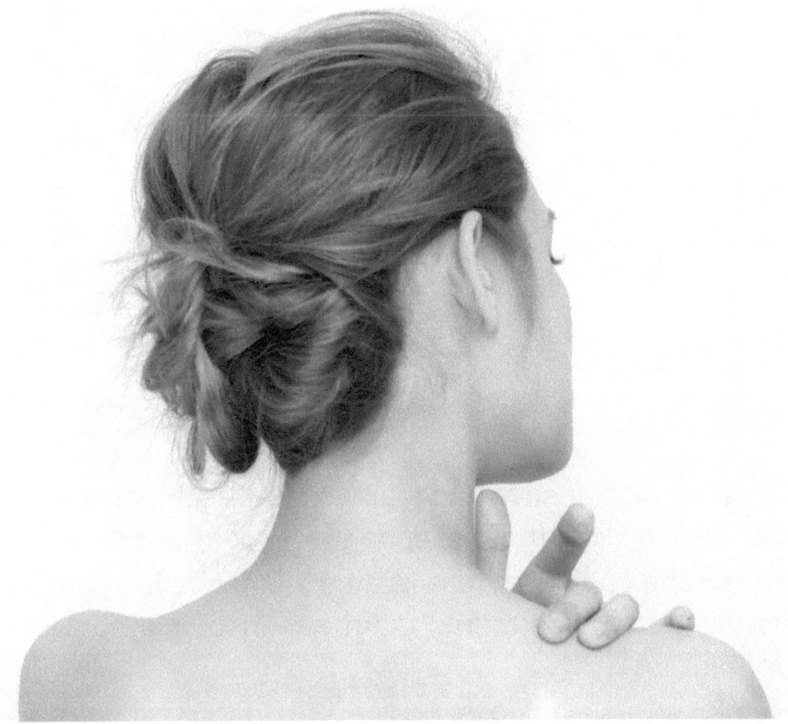

•Helps relieve local pain, headaches, tension, neck pain, shoulder pain, trapezius strain.

•Resolves insubstantial phlegm of the head such as neck lumps, embolic stroke, swollen lymph nodes, tumors.

•Resolves phlegm of chest and breasts such as mastitis, abscess, asthma, dyspnea.

•Moves Qi down as in coughs, hiccough.

•Promotes milk production in lactating women.

•Promotes labor. *Contraindicated during pregnancy

Ren 12-Central Belly/Zhong Wan. Location: Midway between belly button and intercostal angle.

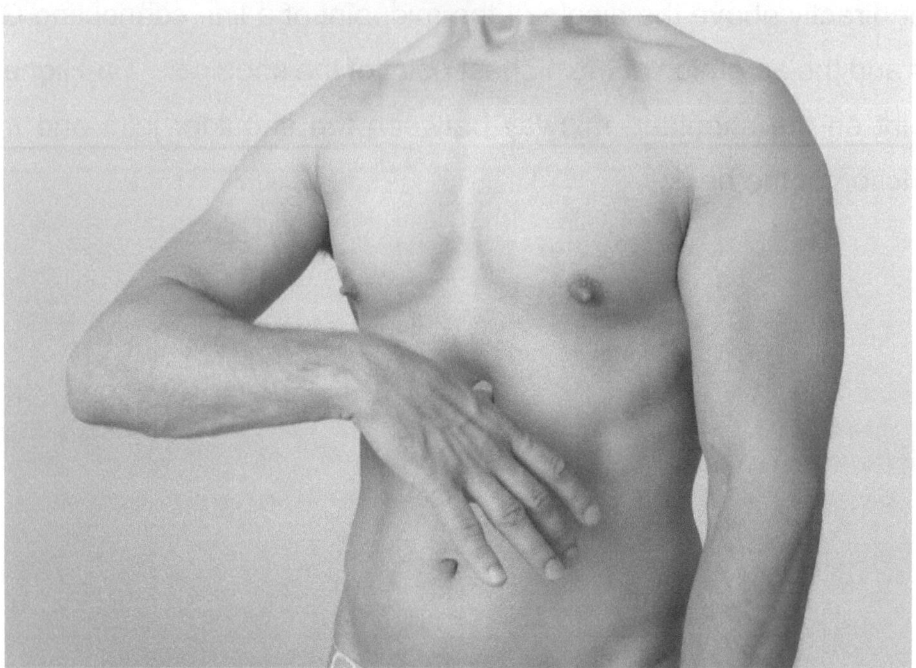

•Good for all digestive and stomach issues, bloating, fullness, reflux, vomiting, diarrhea, esophagus issues, jaundice.
•Boosts the spirit for stress related stomach disorders, IBS, nervous stomach, heartburn, diarrhea, insomnia, anxiety, worry, overthinking.
•Helpful with weight loss.

Seal Hall or Third Eye/Yin Tang. Location: Center between the medial ends of the eyebrows.

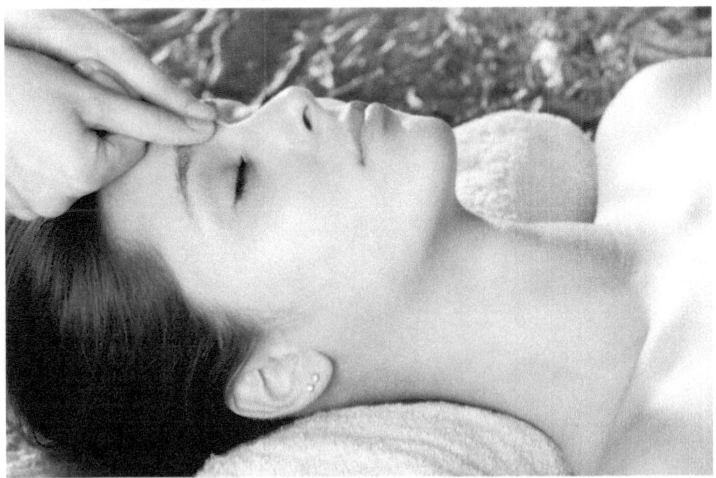

- Insomnia, stress, anxiety
- Frontal headache.
- Sinus congestion, rhinitis.
- Eye problems.

Du 20 One Hundred Meetings/Bai Hui. **Location:** on the crow of the head, on the imaginary line drawn from the tip of the ears t the center of the head. It is considered the meeting place of on hundred spirits.

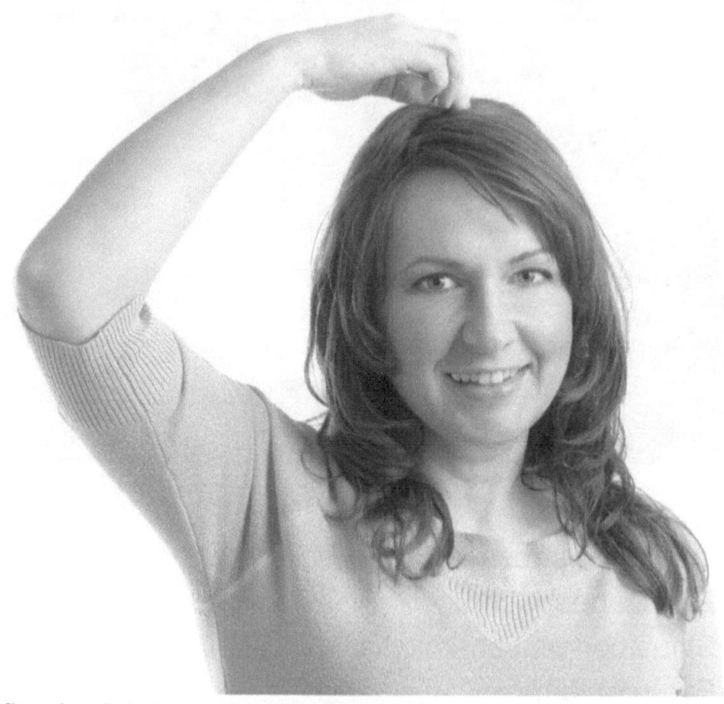

•Benefits the brain and sense organs.
•Lifts organs-helps keep organs in their proper place, prevents prolapses.
•As the opposite pole of the Du meridian, it can treat symptoms relating to the coccyx and perineum.
•Lifts the mood and spirit, mental disorders, depression, and anx-iety.

A Healthy Center

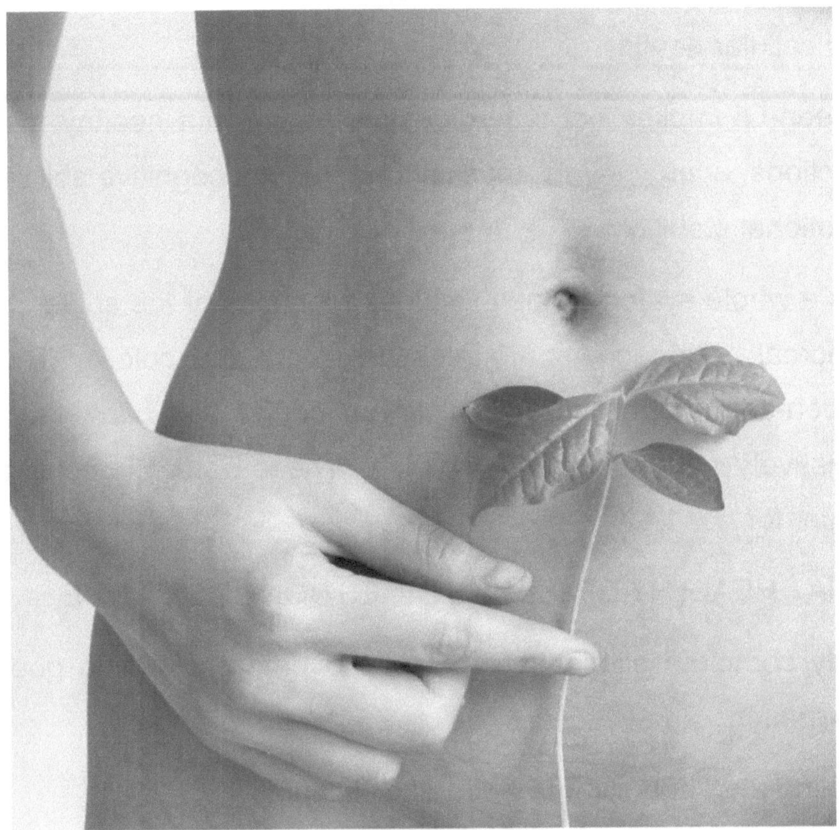

The spleen and stomach meridian systems are responsible

for transforming our food and drink into Qi-energy and blood. The significance is that the spleen transports this energy and blood all over the body to our cells, tissues, and other organs. It also controls blood by holding it in the vessels and taking part in some of the formation of blood. The spleen controls the muscles and limbs and physical energy. The mouth has a functional relationship with the spleen as our sense of taste. Also, the spleen raises the Qi-energy keeping the internal organs in their proper place. Our thought, studying, concentration, thinking clearly, focusing, memorizing are important indicators of spleen health. It can also influence immune and cellular health.

Spleen-Qi implies not only digestive health, but healthy metabolic functions, energy levels, muscle tone, mental cognitive abilities, and emotional stability.

It is a whole system, which includes functions of the spleen, lymph, pancreas, stomach, small intestine, liver, and colon. Thus, the spleen-stomach organ system is our center that can positively or negatively influence everything else. These Earth Elements are the center for health.

WHAT HEALTHY SPLEEN-QI DIGESTION LOOKS LIKE

Daily complete elimination (bowel movement), Feeling good after elimination

Feeling alert and clear headed after eating

Pleasant taste in mouth

Normal body weight, Good muscle tone

Able to work hard, Practical and responsible

Strong, active, stable, Good endurance

Healthy appetite and satisfaction after meals

SYMPTOMS OF POOR SPLEEN-QI DIGESTION, AND TOXIC BUILD UP IN YOUR BODY

Constipation, loose stools or diarrhea, Hemorrhoids

Obesity

Melasma (cholasma): brown to gray-brown patches on skin, usually on the face.

Acne (pimple), black heads

Bad breath

Itchy skin, rashes, eczema

Irritable bowel syndrome, Gas and bloating, tummyache

Nausea or lack of appetite, Ulcers

Headaches, Insomnia, Fatigue

Sugar cravings or cravings for refined carbohydrate foods

Poor focus, memory or concentration, worry, anxiety, obsessiveness

Teeth grinding

Stress, emotional upset, lack of self-control, anger, frustration, depression, irritability.

Allergies and asthma

Arthritis, joint pain, stiffness, difficulty moving the body or limbs

Muscular aches and pains, soreness, muscle fatigue, lack of endurance

Chinese Medicine Dietary Principles

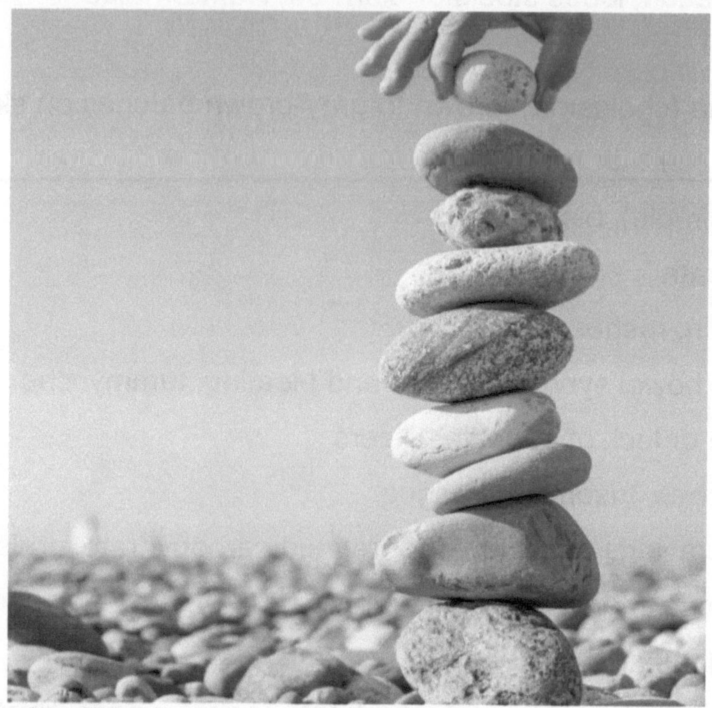

Chinese Medicine has been around for centuries, and the theories and practices still apply to the modern people of today for all populations, and ethnicity.

Follow a balanced diet per Traditional Chinese Medicine (TCM) for a healthy life, called the Spleen-Qi diet. Like the Mediterranean diet, it is mostly plant based, but emphasizes a balance between the five flavors bitter, sweet and bland, spicy, salty, and sour as well as thermal energetic qualities of hot and cold foods.

Food categories such as vegetables and leafy greens, proteins, fruits, essential fats, nuts and seeds, whole grains, fermented foods, sea vegetables and microalgae, empty sweets, spices and herbs, as well as methods of cooking are either recommended or restricted depending on your Meridian body type.

Why does it work?

Keep in mind that the basic metabolic and digestive physiology is the same, and that the basic nutritional requirements are the same for everyone. However, we each respond differently to foods because each person may differ in physical needs and have varying mental and emotional tendencies. Foods, we think are good for us can lead to digestive or other health problems if we are unable to assimilate them properly.

When in good health, most people living in temperate climates do well on the Spleen-Qi diet.

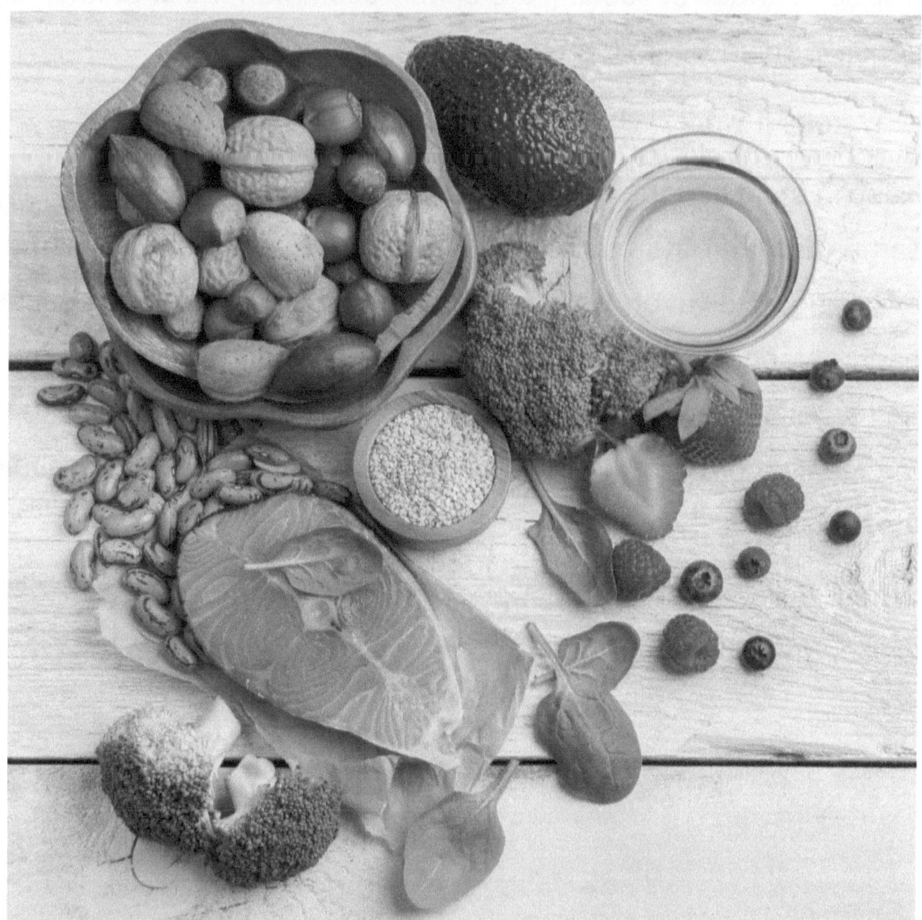

Follow the Healthful Tips Based on the Tradition of Chinese Medicine below. Diet is everything!

TRADITIONAL CHINESE MEDICINE HEALTH RULES

These healthy rules apply to children as well as adults, and they are meant to be followed for a healthy lifestyle.

Minimize or eliminate soda, black tea, milk products, and for adults also exclude coffee, alcohol, and don't smoke.

Follow the 80/20 rule!

Fill your plate with 80% dark leafy greens and vegetables, 20% proteins and good fats.

1. Stop eating when you're 80% full.

2. Eat 3 regular meals each day; develop a routine with 25% food intake at breakfast, 50% at lunch, and 25% at dinner.

3. Take time out for relaxation. Enjoy meals in a calm state, don't eat standing up or while working or reading.

4. Chew food thoroughly, eat slowly, it takes 20 min. for your stomach to know it's full.

5. Most meals should provide a balance of 5 flavors (bitter, sweet-bland, spicy, salty, and sour), natures (warming, cooling, cold, or hot), plus have the array of five colors (red, green, orange-yellow, purple-dark, white-tan). Be sure to vary your types of foods. You don't have to have all food groups, flavors, and colors in one meal, but if you consume 20% from each type of flavor, and color throughout the day you will obtain the most nutrition without eating too much of any one kind.

6. Most meals should be warm. Meals should leave you feeling satisfied but not full. 80% cooked, 20% raw for those with healthy digestive function. For those with poor digestion, keep cold and raw foods to about 5 %.

7. Eat 3:1 ratio of alkalizing foods to acidic forming foods. Coffee, black tea, sugar, meats, milk, and grains are considered

concentrated foods, and are acidic forming. Counteract by eating alkalizing foods such as vegetables and dark leafy greens.

8. Regular sleep patterns; go to bed and wake at the same time every day.

9. Don't eat three hours prior to bedtime.

10. Regular exercise, at least 3-5 times per week. Use a pedometer to record at least 10,000 steps per day equal to 5 miles.

11. Crowd out eating processed refined sugars, high fructose corn syrup, Agave, polyunsaturated vegetable oils, canola oil, safflower oil, cotton seed oil, & grains such as white flour and most white rice products.

12. Eat only organic Non-GMO foods. Consume Non-GMO organic soy only in traditional Asian forms of Tofu, Miso, Tempeh, Natto, or Tamari.

13. Drink plenty of fresh water per day. Add lemon juice or a few drops of lemon essential oil for alkalinity, and increased glutathione levels (antioxidant) to aid in natural cleansing and detoxification, and digestive support. Do not drink large amounts of liquid with meals. Not only does liquid dilute stomach acid and make it harder for your stomach to break down food, it also overwhelms the spleen Qi. It is best to drink a small cup of warm tea, miso soup, or broth with meals than cold iced water.

14. Enjoy the sunshine 2-3 X per week; depending on your skin type, weather, etc. or until your skin turn's lightly pink; don't burn! This is

important for natural vitamin D formation that just can't be beat by vitamins.

15. Reduce stress, find ways to help you deal with stress more effectively, like mediation, Tai Chi, Qi Gong, Yoga, Acupuncture, massage therapy, walking, or other fun hobby.

16. Have regular acupuncture treatments to keep your Qi-energy and Blood flowing smoothly.

The following are general guidelines per the Spleen-Qi Diet of what to eat or not to eat to stay healthy.

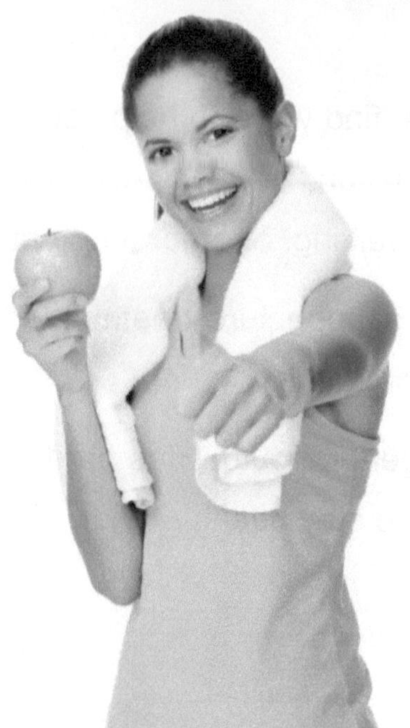

Use only organic, Non-GMO foods, no artificial sweeteners, preservatives, or colors.

Dark Leafy Greens: chard, kale, spinach, parsley, watercress, red leaf lettuce, boy choy, alfalfa sprouts, mustard greens, turnip greens, collard greens, beet greens, seaweeds, and micro-algae (chlorella, spirulina), wheat and barley grasses.

Sea vegetables: Wakame, dulce, kelp, nori, bladderwrack.

Fresh, low starch vegetables: cucumber, broccoli, cauliflower, celery, turnip, radish, onion, green bean, sweet pea, zucchini, leek, garlic, eggplant, bell pepper, mushrooms, asparagus, summer squash, okra.

Plant protein: Lentils, quinoa, edamame (young green soybean).

Animal protein: Grass-fed meats, free-range poultry, and eggs if they aren't a toxic trigger.

Cold-Water Fish, Wild Caught Fish: Atlantic mackerel, cod, haddock, herring, mahi-mahi, salmon, anchovies, pollock, trout, whitefish, canned light tuna and sardines.

Foods for the microflora in your gut: organic raw unpasteurized sauerkraut and its juice, seaweeds (start with 1/2 cup per day, best is unsalted); miso-soy paste, tamari-a gluten free soy sauce (1/2 teaspoon daily-test for intolerance, if so, there will be weakness and tiredness soon after eating); tempeh or tofu, best if cooked; organic naturally brewed, unfiltered, unpasteurized apple cider vinegar. Use 1/3 Cup water mixed with 1 tsp. apple cider vinegar three times per day. Optional to add 1 tsp. raw organic unpasteurized honey. Apple cider vinegar shouldn't be taken with watery stools, or muscular weakness. As you feel improvement, take frequent breaks from this as you don't want to develop a dependency; organic raw unpasteurized yogurt without sugar; kefir, which has three times the number of probiotics than yogurt.

Fats and Oils: Avocado, and its oil, olive oil, ghee (clarified butter), sesame seed and oil, flax seed and oil, coconut milk, coconut oil. Eat in small amounts. Other sources include whole-fat milk, whole-fat yogurt, lean grass-fed beef and pork, whole eggs, olives, parmesan cheese, ricotta cheese, feta cheese, mozzarella cheese, super firm tofu (also provides lots of protein).

Nuts, Seeds, Nut Butters: Almonds, almond butter, walnuts, pista chios, sunflower seeds, sesame seeds, tahini (sesame seed butter pumpkin seeds, chia seeds, hemp seeds. Choose seeds and nut that are in their shells, or lightly roasted and unsalted. Raw nuts g rancid quickly and may harbor parasites.

Fruits: Berries, lemons, limes, pink grapefruit, non-molding fruit such as apples, pears.

Foods with anti-fungal properties: Coconut oil, cinnamon, tur meric, onion, garlic, olives, olive oil, foods rich in omega 3 fatty acids Olives and olive oil contain a chemical compound, oleuropein, whicl doesn't allow Candida to thrive.

Simple sugars: Stevia, organic Non-GMO unrefined cane sugar unprocessed organic unpasteurized honey. Honey has naturally oc curring digestive enzymes and minerals. Real 100% maple syrup Use empty sweets sparingly.

Salts: Unprocessed sea-salt, seaweed salts used sparingly.

Beverages: Green Tea, Fresh filtered water (not distilled).

Foods to Crowd-Out Summary

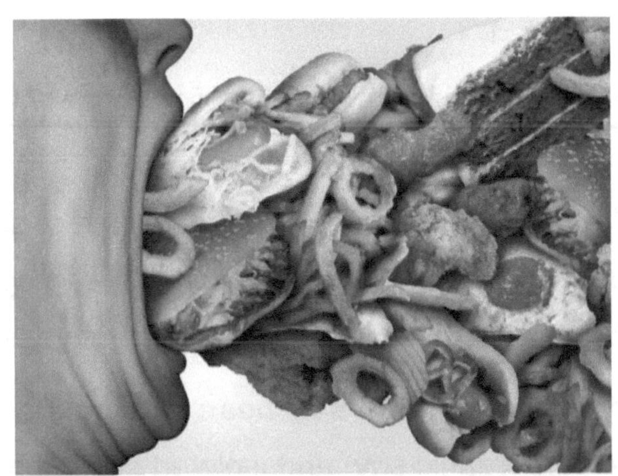

Crowd out unhealthy foods, or foods believed to be toxic triggers for you or your child.

Unhealthy foods: processed foods, refined white sugar, white flour products, bagels, muffins, donuts, cake, pies, cookies, crackers, bread, cereals, granola, candy, milk chocolate, fried, greasy foods, GMO foods.

Most Dairy products: processed cheese, cottage cheese, cream cheese, ice cream, cow's milk, lower fat skim milk, non-fat milk products, non-dairy creamers, commercial yogurt and yogurt with sugar, preservatives, artificial sweeteners. *Do your own research on web or YouTube about how milk and milk products are processed to remove the fats. Today the process is highly mechanized and involves the addition of powdered milk solids. These solids contain oxidized cholesterol, and denatured proteins, both of which contribute to inflammation and plaque buildup. Additionally, the fat in milk is needed for your body to absorb and assimilate the fat-soluble vitamins, D, A,

E, and K. Therefore, adding these vitamins to non-fat milk product doesn't make sense because you won't be able to utilize them anyway.

Processed or fatty meats: Cold cuts, hot dogs, and those foods and meats with sulfites.

Fermented foods: processed with yeast, sugar, or glutinous grains yeasted breads, brewer's yeast, common white vinegar, soy sauce kombucha because it can contain wild strains of yeast.

Soy: soy beans, soy milk, soy bean oil, isolated soy protein Avoid GMO, non-organic soy, and isolated soy in processed foods and in forms not properly prepared as in traditional Asian cuisine.

Rice white or brown (unless organic, Non-GMO). Basmati or Jasmine rice are best.

Peanuts, peanut butter.

Drinks: Alcohol, caffeine, coffee, black tea, soft drinks-especially diet.

Simple Sugars: Refined white cane sugar, brown sugar, powdered sugar, turbinado sugar, raw sugar, syrup, high fructose corn syrup, pasteurized honey, agave because it is highly processed with chemicals. *turbinado, and raw sugar are not unrefined cane sugar. It must say this on the label.

The best empty sweets to choose are unrefined cane sugar (the least processed), 100% maple syrup, Manuka honey, raw unpasteurized honey, black-strap molasses, malt barley, and rice syrup.

Processed iodized table salt.

Foods known to be allergenic or toxic triggers for you. If these foods are thought to be a problem for you avoid them: eggs, fish, shellfish, strawberries, nuts, peanuts, legumes, milk, milk products, soy milk, soy products, or other.

Gluten: If you have Celiac sprue, or celiac disease, allergy, or intolerance to gluten, avoid Wheat, barley, spelt, rye, or glutenous grain. Oats may be alright for some people, if they are labeled certified gluten free. Also, soy sauce may contain wheat. Try a gluten free tamari variety.

Beans and Legumes May be difficult for some people to digest and may depend on the variety or whether they're prepared correctly. They are high in protein and fiber and have many benefits if they're not a toxic trigger for you.

The Nightshades: potatoes, tomatoes, bell peppers, eggplant, onion, garlic, corn, and beets. Some people feel an exacerbation of joint pain or arthritis with the consumption of nightshades.

Harmonize the Liver and Gall Bladder

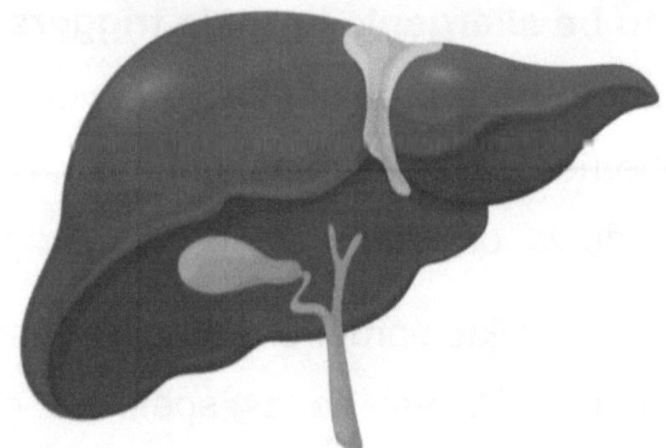

The first remedy is to eat less.

Foods to Avoid are those high in saturated fats, Lard, Mamma meats, Cream, Cheese, Eggs

Avoid Hydrogenated and poor-quality fats, Shortening, Margarine

Avoid Refined and rancid oils

Excess nuts and seeds. They should be unsalted, and lightly roasted. Raw nuts easily become rancid, and harbor parasites.

Chemicals in foods and water

Processed foods

All intoxicants

Eat foods or herbs that stimulate the flow of liver-Qi energy

1. Moderately pungent foods, spices and herbs: watercress, onion, mustard greens, turmeric, basil, bay leaf, cardamom, marjoram, cumin, fennel, dill, ginger, black pepper, horseradish, rosemary, mints, lemon balm (Melissa), angelica (dang gui).

2. Don't eat too much fiery peppers.

3. Others: beets, taro root, sweet rice, amazake, strawberry, peach, cherry, chestnut, pine nut, vegetables of the Brassica genus-cabbage, turnip root, kohlrabi, cauliflower, broccoli, and Brussels sprouts. You may find it easier to digest these when they are lightly cooked, steamed, or stir fried. If you are not used to eating these begin with small amounts and use the spices mentioned above to aid digestion. I cannot emphasize enough the use of those spices!

4. Although alcohol temporarily moves liver energy, it ultimately causes cellular destruction. Avoid it.

5. Eat raw sprouted grains, sprouted beans, sprouted seeds.

6. Raw, organic, unpasteurized honey, used sparingly, is detoxifying. Mix 1 tsp. with 1 tsp. raw organic unpasteurized apple cider vinegar, 1 drop cinnamon essential oil or ½ tsp. cinnamon powder, and 1/3 cup warm water.

*Note: This should not be used as the sole remedy for detoxification, digestive health, or liver function. If you wish to continue apple cider vinegar or the drink, it's best not to develop a dependency. Take periodic breaks for 5 days, every 10 days.

7. The Chinese Medicine herbal formula **Xiao Yao Wan** (Rambling Powder) moves and nourishes the liver energy, and emotional constraint. Ingredients: Bupleurum (Chai Hu), Angelica Root (Dang Gui), White Peony (Bai Shao), White Atractylodes (Bai Zhu), Poria Mushroom (Fu Ling), Honey Baked Licorice (Zhi Gan Cao), Mint (Bo

He), Fresh Ginger (Sheng Jiang). Citrus Peel (Chen Pi), Amomum Cardamom Seed (Sha Ren) can be added for a weak spleen-stomach.

Take twice daily before meals.

Contraindications: Do not take during an acute phase of colds and flu.

Caution: This formula has been modified to reduce likelihood of stomach bloating or loose stools with the additions of Chen Pi and Sha Ren. Should this occur with the additions, take with food, or discontinue.

8.   Licorice root and Chrysanthemum tea can help with the initial stages of detoxification.

9.   Bitter foods to eat include romaine lettuce, asparagus, quinoa, alfalfa, radish leaves, and citrus peel.

10. Seaweeds, kelp, mung beans sprouts, mushrooms, radish, daikon radish, rhubarb root.

11. Fresh cold-pressed flax oil, borage oil, evening primrose oil, black current seed oil.

12. Chlorophyll rich foods: dark grapes, blackberries, huckleberries, raspberries, blackstrap molasses, spirulina, wild blue-green algae, chlorella, parsley, kale, collard greens.

13. Reduce or eliminate sources of toxins such as additives to household and personal care products, insecticides, etc.

14. Use 3 – 5 drops of a **detoxification essential oil blend** applied to liver area daily. Note: A detoxification Blend you can purchase may include Clove, Geranium, Grapefruit and Rosemary, or in a roller ball combine 4 drops **Geranium**, 6 drops **Rosemary**, 6 drops **Cilantro,** 8 drops **Juniper Berry**, and fill remainder with FCO.

*Note: most liver conditions have developed over long periods of time and rebuilding will take consistent application with patience over weeks and months.

-Time frame for a liver cleanse: can be taken indefinitely daily or as a periodic cleanse for 2 weeks every three months.

Alternative liver detoxification Choices

-1 tablespoon of organic Lemon juice daily with water.

-1 drop each of **Lemon** and **Peppermin**t essential oils applied over liver area.

-1 drop **Coriander** essential oils if necessary, for addictions applied over liver area.

-2-4 ounces of purified water daily, drink first thing in the morning.

-Topically apply 2 – 5 drops of **Myrrh** across the back (about the bra line for ladies) daily.

-Basic daily supplements for balanced nutrition as a foundation. Note: Basic daily Supplements include an omega 3 complex from marine and land sources, a whole-food based nutrient and mineral complex, and a cellular vitality complex; For adults who can't take

capsules use the children's chewable tablets and children's liqui
omega3 daily.

-Consider these additional points:

-Sufficient hydration with 1 – 2 drops of **Grapefruit** or **Lemon** adde
to each glass of water.

-Periodic massage using a **Massage Blend** will promote homeosta
sis.   The blend includes basil, grapefruit, cypress, marjoram
lavender, and peppermint.

Gall Bladder Health

Gall Bladder Flush to purge stones or sediment with a one-day ritual

1. Start in the morning and throughout the day, eat only green organic apples-at least 4 or 5.

2. Drink water or herbal teas, apple juice.

3. At bedtime-warm up 2/3 Cup extra virgin olive oil to body temperature, mix in 1/3 cup fresh lemon juice. Slowly sip mixture, then immediately go to bed, lying on right side, with right leg drawn up.

4. In the morning the stones should have passed in the stool

5. Or use a milder, less effective version of the flush over 5 days. Ingest on empty stomach 2 tbsp. olive oil followed by 2 tbsp. fresh lemon juice.

Gradual Gallbladder Cleanse

1. For 21 days eat 1-2 radishes between meals, drink 3 cups cleavers, or 5 cups chamomile tea each day.

2. At one meal each day pour 5 tsp. fresh cold-pressed flax oil over your food, or 2.5 tsp. over your food for 2 meals.

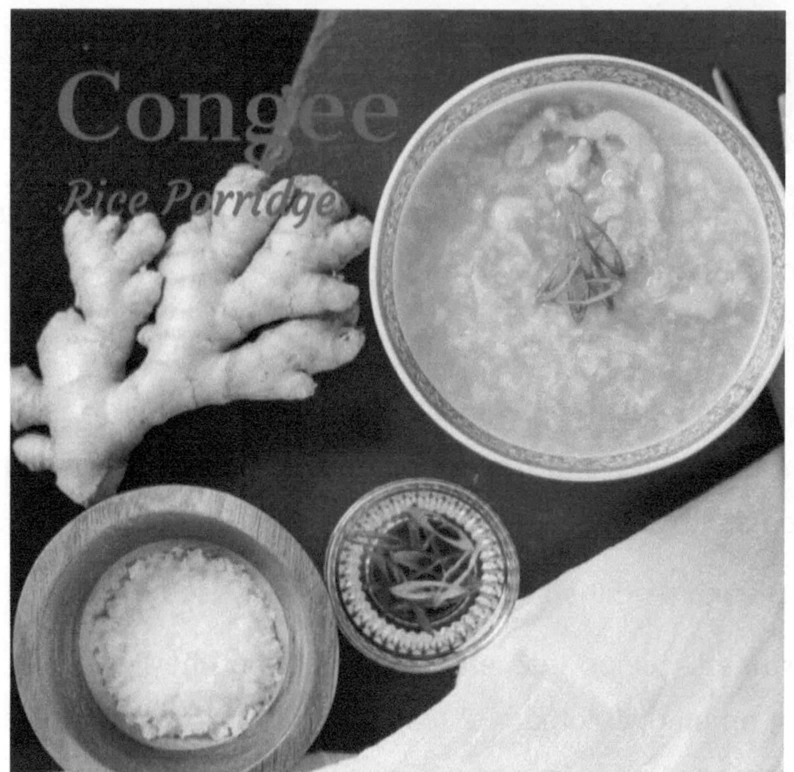

Congee is eaten throughout China as a thin soup or thicker gruel. Generally, you add 3-6 times the amount of liquid to rice, depending on the desired thickness. I use medium or long grain rice, but you can also use short grain. It takes about 1 cup rice to 6 cups or 9 cups liquid. You can always add more liquid if you need to. Use less if you prefer it thicker. Traditionally water is used, but for more flavor you can use broth. You can also use any other grain besides rice. Ideally, you would cook the congee for up to 4-6 hours on low heat; a crockpot works very well for congees. It is said that the longer a congee cooks the "more powerful" it becomes. However, you may find that 25 minutes is enough.

A congee is easily digested, and the nutrients are easily assimilated, thus it fortifies the blood, and Qi-energy, strengthens the Spleen-pancreas digestive-Qi, harmonizes digestion, is moistening, cooling, and nourishing. The liquid can be strained to drink as a supplement for infants or for those with serious illness. By itself, rice cooked with water is very bland. This is best for infants, or when ill or recuperating from illness or surgery. Other desired therapeutic benefits for food therapy can be achieved by the addition of appropriate vegetables, grains, meats, or herbs. It can be made with foods for their cooling effects or more warming effects.

The addition of garnishes or toppings add color, texture and taste. Try hard boiled eggs, mussels, clams, nuts, seeds, fried shallots, fresh herbs, cilantro, basil, green onion, chive, celery, fish sauce, chili paste, a drizzle of tamari, or sesame oil. It can be seasoned with white or black pepper, sea salt, ginger slices, minced garlic, sea vegetables, pickled greens, or pickled vegetables. For breakfast, or a sweeter taste try cinnamon, nutmeg, clove, red dates, goji berries, fresh blue berries, maple syrup, barley or rice malt. You can choose to sauté garlic, ginger and mushrooms in olive, sesame, or avocado oil until mushrooms have softened before adding the rice and liquid. Stir in greens and other quick cooking vegetables in the last hour or minutes of cooking time. It can stay refrigerated for a few days. If it thickens while in the refrigerator, add an appropriate amount of broth or water when reheating.

Ancient Healing for Modern People

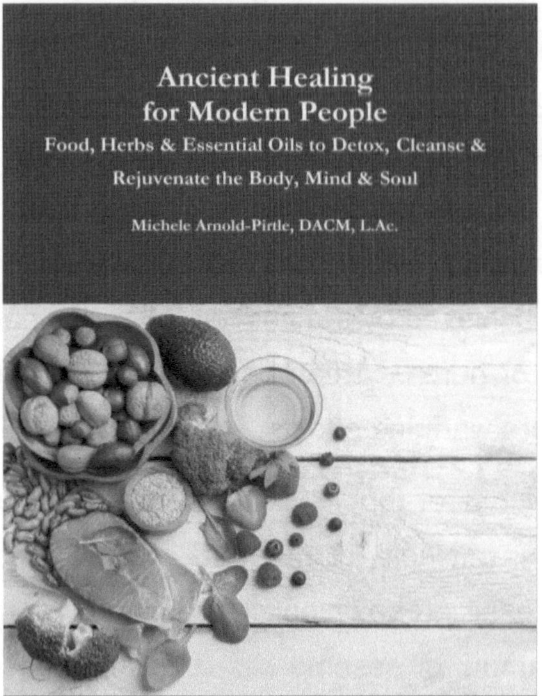

More details, and recipes are included in the book, "Ancient Healing for Modern People: Food, Herbs & Essential Oils to Detox, Cleanse & Rejuvenate the Body, Mind & Soul", By Michele Arnold-Pirtle, DACM, L.Ac.

Use Chinese Medicine Dietary Principles for a gentle yet effective way to detox and cleanse your body and gut. For in depth details about Chinese Medicine, and the best dietary practices with food, herbs, and essential oils.

It can be found on Amazon and Lulu.com. Available in print or eBook. There are print copies for sale at Acupuncture Center, Inc.

This book is designed to be used by both laypeople as well as holistic health practitioners and acupuncturists. This can serve as a resource and guide for dietary guidelines and suggestions per individual constitutional Meridian body types.

It covers how to do a 10-day essential body detox and gut restoration program, with a 10-day menu plan, and provides details about a healthy Spleen-Qi Diet.

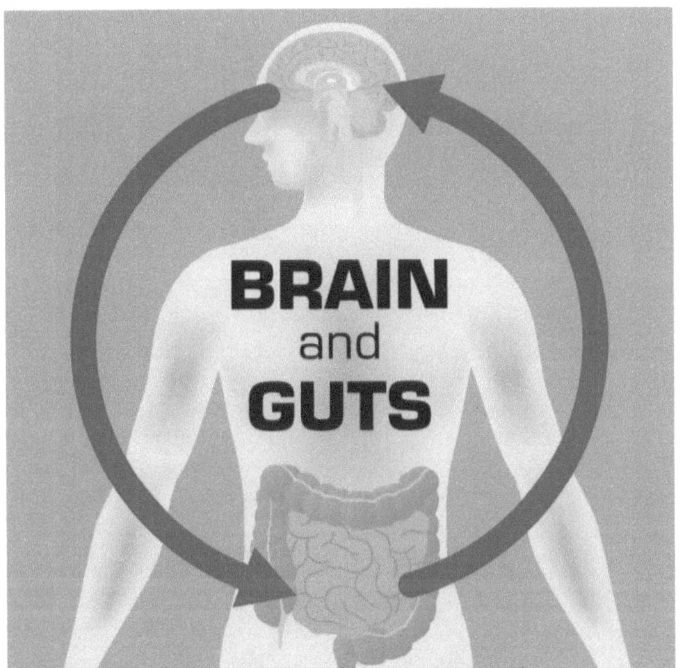

Western science along with Chinese Medicine both confirm that a healthy gut is necessary for our immune systems. In addition, there are more neurons in our gut than our brain, and we also know the gut and its hormones affects our brain, emotions, and behavior.

The musculoskeletal system depends on healthy digestion for movement and relaxation. Our digestive systems extract the vital nutrients we need from our food and drink to nourish our joints, bones, and muscles.

Continue with a healthy Spleen-Qi (balanced) diet or a diet plan per your Meridian body type for long-term health and vitality.

Less Stress Improves Your Health

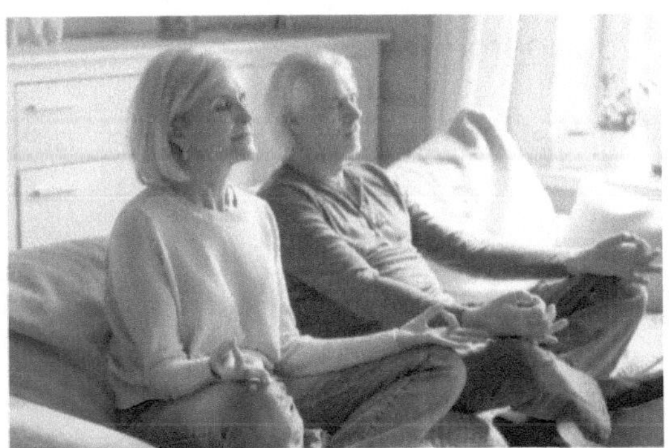

Why is reducing stress, and enhancing one's spiritual-emotional well-being so important to your health?

Stress disturbs our energetic balance by generating dysfunction and weakening the body. How can we learn to react, and handle daily stresses more appropriately? One way is by enhancing one's emotional-spiritual well-being. First, let's describe what is the meaning of spirituality.

Spiritualty is our belief system, and core values. Spirituality encompasses the following ideas:

1. Meaning and purpose of life

2. Relationships with other people, and the universe

3. Existence of a higher power, and your relationship with them

4. Past lives

5. After-lives

6. Meaning of hardship, suffering and tribulations

7. impermanence of our lives, aging, disease, and death.

Your health, wealth, and happiness are determined by your virtue or bad-karma. Virtues or bad-karma affects your outlook:

1. Determines your perception of life's events

2. This perception determines your emotional, behavioral, and physical reactions.

3. Subsequently affects body's energy, biochemistry, and structural makeup.

4. Therefore, maintaining spiritual-emotional well-being is essential to your health, mentally and physically.

To cultivate spiritual health is Life Cultivation!

Qi-Gong, Tai-Chi, mediation are forms of life cultivation systems.

Apply truthfulness, compassion, and endurance in life, which will return you to your true-self. Begin with the four steps below that will reduce stress levels by enhancing your spiritual-emotional well-being.

1. Begin by practicing Self-Love and Kindness towards yourself. This allows you to be present instead of trying to escape into the future or staying in the past.

2. Focus on your sense of purpose. This doesn't have to be a big thing, nor do you need to save the world.

What are you supposed to be doing on this Earth? Why are you here? Don't make it complicated. Remind yourself of your PURPOSE every, single, day. Having a focus gives you something to focus on and something to do.

3. Express gratitude for EVERYTHING. Be grateful and learn how to focus on gratitude.

With gratitude comes simplicity which gives you the ability to simplify. Gratitude helps you to realize that you really don't have a problem right now in the grand scheme of things.

Reframing your outlook into a sense of gratitude for the opportunity to be here on this planet, to be here in this moment, in this physical, mental, spiritual place with all the beautiful things around you.

4. Enjoy, and be thankful for the miracle of the life around you. The air, the ability to breathe...the colors...the plants...the warm sun...cool nights...fresh water...the birds...the pets...the people...and more!

To live is an OPPORTUNITY.

Five aspects of our lives, biological, social-behavioral, psychological, spiritual, and financial are affected by 3 levels of existence. The 3 levels of existence are:

1. Structural

2. Chemical

3. Energetic

Many severe illnesses or disease begin at the energetic level before they are detectable by modern medical science. They may even stay at that level causing a significant amount of suffering and disability.

Many can agree that amazing progress has been made by modern medicine taking care of the structural and bio-chemical components of disease.

Acupuncture and Chinese Medicine takes care of the human energy system, and it is a crucial part in integrative medicine.

For instance, in acute trauma to a person's low back and leg from a skiing accident, the muscles, ligaments, tendons, and bones may be involved. This may be noticed by the naked-eye clinically, or by an X-ray machine. However, there are also bio-chemical reactions and inflammation taking place as well. These may be noticed via scientific laboratory examination of the person's blood sample.

There is also an energetic interruption of the Qi-energy meridian system causing pain or illness. Although invisible, the meridians are essential to keep the body functioning and alive. If we don't recognize the energetic patterns of dysfunction at the meridian level, and treat accordingly, we are not able to heal the patient effectively, and entirely.

Western Medicine uses heroic, and drastic treatments like chemotherapy, radiation, pharmaceutical medications, or surgery. These may be helpful to treat structural, bio-chemical or physiological symptoms, but they can generate unwanted side-effects due to their negative effect on the meridian system.

Acupuncture can help reduce side-effects and enhance the outcomes of conventional therapies. Acupuncture can detect energetic disruptions and provide a clinical picture for understanding the disharmony. Energetic homeostasis is when people can feel their emotions as situationally appropriate, and feel content, and even-keeled most of the time.

Natural Blood Thinners and Pain Reducers

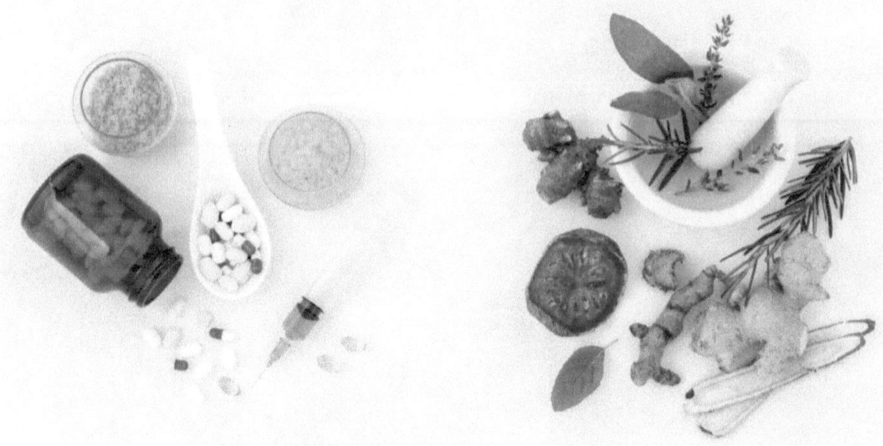

The phenomenon of acute and chronic pain has fueled multimillion-dollar industries for aspirin, acetaminophen, opioid containing drugs, steroids, and other analgesics. Aspirin is known to improve cardiovascular health and the patency of blood flow in the vessels, as well as working as an effective pain reliever. Chronic use of these drugs comes with a price, however. To reap the benefits of aspirin, is like borrowing from Peter to pay Paul. This is because aspirin works by suppressing the body's natural inflammatory reaction. Aspirin and various steroid drugs block the production of a type of prostaglandin, PGE 2, therefore reducing blood clotting, fever, and pain. The downfall is that it also blocks production of the type PGE 1. Though it works to reduce symptoms, behind the scenes inflammation and tissue deterioration from arthritis and heart disease continues from higher leukotrienes. Consumption of excess animal products contributes excessive amounts of arachidonic acid (AA). The AA not only encourages production of PGE 2, but leukotrienes as well. Leukotrienes are beneficial in wound healing, but in high amounts not controlled by natural anti-inflammatory reactions they may provoke breast lumps, and arthritis. PGE 1 has its own anti-inflammatory properties and increases in PGE1 and 3 limits production of PGE 2 and leukotrienes. A diet rich in omega-3 fatty acids can be helpful to keep these chemicals in proper balance.

The major component of aspirin is salicylic acid, which has widespread metabolic effects. Taking over a long period of time can damage the kidneys. It also increases bleeding tendencies and can cause stomach bleeding. It is not recommended for those with diabetes, kidney or liver disease, or ulcers. It triples the excretion of vitamin C. These negative effects are especially enhanced if aspirin is taken more than the conservative approach of one tablet every other day. To benefit the cardiovascular system aspirin can negatively affect other systems. Fortunately, there are safer natural alternatives.

Food Therapy for Improved Blood Flow

1. A diet high in vitamin A, C, B complex vitamins and calcium-rich foods. Sources may include carrots, eggs, liver, dark leafy greens.

2. Limit excessive consumption of animal products. Although grass-fed animals and their dairy products are high in omeg-3s, they are still highly concentrated with AA and PGE 2. Instead use omega-3s from Alpha-linolenic acid from flax, chia, pumpkin seeds, dark green

plants. Also, Gamma-linoleic acid is produced by your body from linolenic acid. It can also be found directly from spirulina, borage seed oil, black current seed oil, and evening primrose seed oil. Fatty cold-water fish such as tuna, sardine, salmon, anchovy, or fish oi can provide sources of EPA and DHA omega-3s.

3. Improve posture and spine health. Try the 90/90 solution: lie or the floor, legs on a chair, with the legs at a 90-degree angle. Alternatively, you can lie on your side in the same position. As you lie keep your arms outstretched to the side, and your head straight Breath slowly, and from the lower abdomen. Slowly move your head looking to the left, then center, then right, and back to center. Try to keep the position for 20 minutes. Roll slowly to your side, and then ease yourself up.

4. Avoid nitrate, and MSG, containing foods, and reduce caffeine consumption. Foods generally higher in nitrates may include chocolate, coca, and luncheon meats. Slowly ease yourself off caffeine to avoid a withdrawal headache.

5. **Use ice and heat.** Soothe aches and pain initially with an ice pack for 10-15 minutes, then apply heat for 15-20 minutes.

Rub it in! Use a Pain Killing Essential Oil Blend

Where to buy

Essential oil blends and aromatherapy can be purchased from your acupuncturist, holistic health practitioner, or aromatherapist.

Higher quality brands can be ordered on-line through your provider, or you can set up your own whole-sale account as a customer through an essential oil representative.

How to use

Apply to affected area every 20-30 minutes for acute pain, reducing frequency as pain is reduced.

For chronic conditions apply 2-3 times per day. For those with skin sensitivities reduce or stop use if skin irritation occurs. Here are 2 examples of effective essential oil remedies. Add oil drops to 5-ml. roller bottle or small glass bowl, then fill remainder with a carrier oil such as sesame oil, olive oil, grapeseed oil, or fractionated coconut oil (FCO).

-Warming Blend: Copaiba 10 drops, Ginger 10 drops, rosemary 5 drops, peppermint 5 drops, black pepper 5 drops.

-Cooling Blend: Copaiba 10 drops, Marjoram 5 drops, peppermint 5 drops, lavender 10 drops, basil 5 drops.

Chinese herbal teas for pain relieving & muscle relaxing qualities

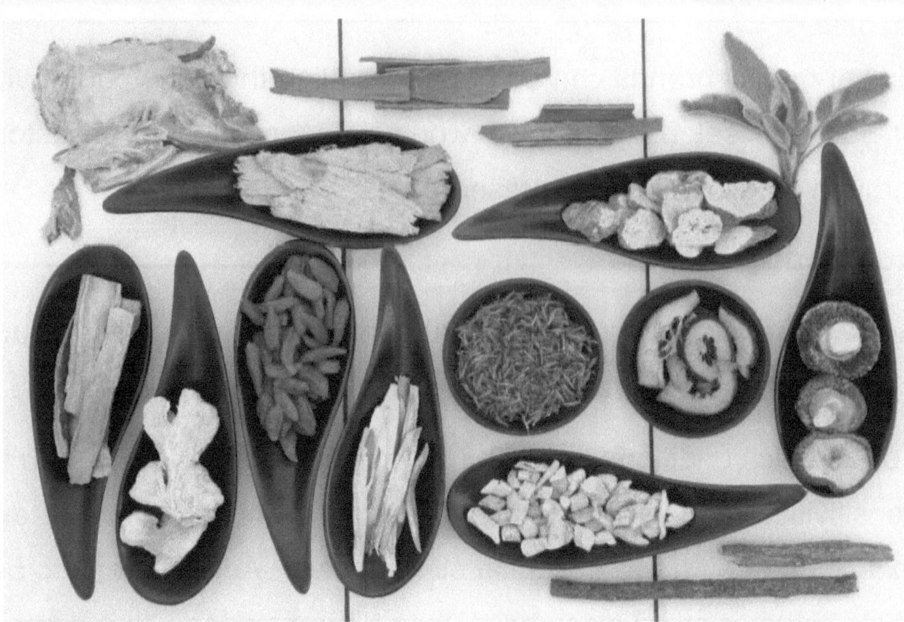

Chinese Herbal Teas are concentrated granules of raw herbal ingredients boiled in an aqueous solution. They are free from preservatives, additives, and colors. They are certified pharmaceutical grade using GMP (Good Manufacturing Practices). The powder is mixed with warm water and drunk as a medicinal tea.

They also come in other forms of administration such as honey pills, capsules, tablets, or alcohol or glycerin extracted tinctures.

Where to buy

Herbal Formulas can be prescribed and purchased from your local Acupuncturist.

Xue Fu Zhu Yu Tang (Drive out Stasis in the Mansion of Blood Decoction).

TCM Diagnosis: Blood stagnation, especially of the upper body, head and chest.

Action: Nourishes and moves blood, a natural analgesic alternative.

Indications: Pain Acute, Severe, after Trauma, aggravated by wrong movement, fixed localized pain, occasional stabbing pain aggravated by certain postures or movement, and pain is worse at night, a natural alternative to aspirin.

Bio-medical or common disease names: acute endometritis, retained placenta, pelvic inflammatory disease, endometriosis, cirrhosis of the liver, intestinal obstruction, coronary artery disease, angina pectoris, rheumatic valvular heart disease, hypertension, post-concussion syndrome, migraine, menopausal syndrome, urticaria, psychosis.

Ingredients: Dang Gui (Chinese Angelica), Chuan Xiong (Szechuan Lovage Root), Sheng Di Huang (Prepared Rehmannia), Chi Shao (Red Peony), Tao Ren (Peach Pit), Hong Hua (Safflower), Chuan Niu Xi (Cyathula Root), Jie Geng (Platycodon, Balloon Flower Root), Zhi Ke (Bitter Orange Peel), Chai Hu (Bupleurum, Thorowax Root), Gan Cao (Licorice Root). Plus add turmeric-curcumin (Yu Jin), cinnamon bark (Rou Gui), Bai Shao (White Peony), and Gan Cao (Licorice).

How to Take: Take Before meals. In severe cases can increases dosage 50-100%, then reduced as treatment takes effect.

Contraindications/Cautions:

Contraindicated in pregnancy, excessive menstrual bleeding, bleeding diathesis, or hemorrhagic disorder. For women, stop taking during your period unless otherwise directed. Caution in patient taking anti-coagulants.

*Women being treated for menstrual problems may notice heavier more painful periods, expulsion of clots, for one or two cycles as the stagnation is moved, and they are encouraged to continue formula for several cycles.

Modifications

Psychological-Emotional herbal additions

-Psychosis, insomnia: Yu Jin (Curcuma), Yuan Zhi (Platycodon), He Huan Pi (Albizzia), Dan Shen (Salvia); for manic behavior add Long Gu (dragon bone), and Mu Li (oyster shell).

-Heart Blood Stasis from anger, frustration, resentment, excess joy, shock, craving, guilt: Xue Fu Zhu Yu Tang

-Anxiety, restless, insomnia, depression, heart palpitations, mood swings, irritability, waking frequently at night, tossing and turning with nightmares, possible chest pain, tongue is purple: Add Shi Chang Pu (Acori), and Yu Jin (Curcuma).

-Liver Blood Stasis from anger, frustration, hate, jealousy, guilt, Emotional-Mental symptoms: extreme depression, mood swings, intense irritability, violent angry outbursts, obsessive jealousy, manic behavior: Add Yu Jin (Curcuma), He Huan Pi (Albizzia) and Suan Zao Ren (Ziziphus).

-Blood stasis in lower burner; Tai-yang organ with blood congestion from anger, frustration, hatred, resentment, guilt or the following-

-Mental-emotional: psychosis following child birth, fever at night, delirium, severe lower abdominal pain, mental restlessness, manic behavior: Tao He Chen Qi Wan with Da Huang (Rhubarb) and Mang Xiao (Mirabilite, sodium sulfate).

Gynecology

Endometriosis, fibroids, adhesions, cysts from Liver Blood Stasis & Phlegm in uterus: add Gui Zhi Fu Ling Wan (Cinnamon Twig & Poria).

Alternative Formula-Gui Zhi Tang (Cinnamon Twig for Analgesia)

Ingredients: cinnamon (Gui Zhi), white peony (Bai Shao), fresh ginger (Sheng Jiang), and red jujube/dates (Da Zao). Plus, the addition of Ge Gen (Pueria, Kudzu Root), Qiang Huo (Notopterygium), Gan Cao (Licorice), Yi-Yi Ren (Coicis-Job's tears or Chinese Pearl Barley are gluten-free), and Fu Ling (Poria mushroom).

Presentation and Indications as an analgesic: pain worse with rest, stiffness, spasms, contracted muscles, tendons, chronic bronchitis, poor immunity, torticollis, stiff neck & upper back.

How to Take:

-Best taken warm after a meal, TID (three X per day). Follow dosage guidelines. Average adult single dose is 3g mixed with 1/4 c or more of warm water. Mix well. Once slight sweating occurs you can stop taking the formula if you are taking it for a common cold.

*Using spoon provided, 1 level spoonful equals approx. 1 gram.

*Empty capsules each are approx. equal to .5 gram, thus 6 capsules are about 3 g for one dose. Swallow with warm water.

-Options: Can mix with rice congee (gruel), porridge.

-Avoid alcohol, cold, greasy, spicy, raw foods during medication.

-Appropriate for after childbirth, or after serious illness. Safe for long term use except as contraindicated below.

Contraindications/Cautions:

-With profuse sweating.

-Use caution in warm weather, summer heat, with high fever, sore throat-unless properly modified for wind-heat. Modifications to clear heat examples may include Huang Qin (Scutellaria), Shi Gao (Gypsum), Zhi Mu (Anemarrhena), Bo He (mint).

-Use with caution when there is hypertension or hemorrhagic disease. Use caution with diuretic drugs.

Why Use CBD (Cannabinoid) Oil?

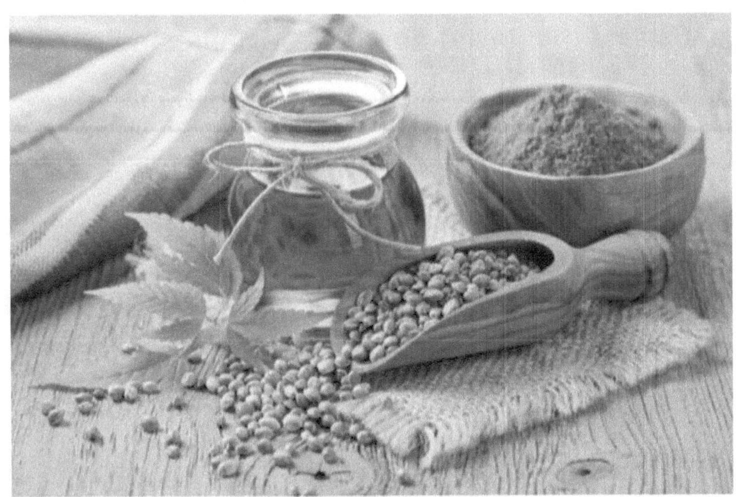

CBD oil has been shown clinically, and via research to aid the body in reducing pain, stress, controlling seizures, balance the CNS, and improve sleep functions. This occurs via the human endocannabinoid system. Cannabinoids and cannabidiol (CBD) from the hemp plant are analogous to the naturally occurring neurotransmitters endocannabinoids of the human body.

The endocannabinoid system is linked to our brain, nervous system, immune system, and digestive system. There are endocannabinoid receptors throughout the body such as the brain, central nervous system, peripheral nervous system, immune system and epidermis.

Benefits of CBD with Zero THC (Tetrahydrocannabinol) or Less Than 0.03% THC

This is equal to 99.99%, considered trace amounts or THC free. No failed drug tests, and it can't get you high.

No fear of mind-altering affects.

Complies with the guidelines of the Substance Abuse and Mental Health Services Administration (SAMHSA).

You may feel calm, relaxed and less anxious, and even drowsy, but not high. You would have to consume quite a lot.

The average CBD user takes between 1/mg a day and 40/mg. At that rate, it would be almost impossible to fail a drug test because of THC.

*Note-if the CBD makes you feel drowsy, take it only before bedtime. Everyone responds differently, and not everyone feels the sedative effect. However, it may balance the circadian rhythm, improving sleep cycles.

Benefits include:

- Natural pain relief and anti-inflammation effects

- Used to treat epilepsy

- Anxiety

- Digestive issues

- Trouble sleeping and insomnia

- Irritated skin – Acne

- Support for Cancer, nausea, and pain.

Ways to use it include:

Tinctures-Take ¼, ½, 1 or 2 droppers per day under the tongue. The amount depends on the concentration level of CBD in the tincture, the degree of pain or discomfort, and how much you find you need to reach desired results. Follow directions on the package.

Edible Gummies-Consume 1 Gummy as needed, before bedtime, or twice dally with morning and evening routine.

Topicals-Creams, salves, massage lotion. Use as needed, or twice daily with morning and evening routine.

Vaporizing-Vape 1-3 times per day.

Capsules-As prescribed or recommended for slower extended release. Follow directions on the package.

Where to buy it

You can find Hemp CBD Oil from your acupuncturist or other holistic health provider. These are not medical marijuana dispensaries. They don't carry the kind of cannabis that gets you high. Therefore, you don't need a medical marijuana card, referral or prescription.

There are two sources of CBD oil. One source is the hemp plant, while the other comes from the marijuana plant.

These two sources vary in their genetic makeup and the purpose for which people grow them. Hemp has been grown and bred to contain little to no THC. Products considered CBD oil, THC free must come from the, "Industrialized hemp plant". CBD from Industrialized Hemp is free from the THC psychoactive constituent.

Marijuana plants contain a higher level of THC, which is a psychoac tive drug that binds to the endocannabinoid system's cannabinoid receptors. It's the agent inside of marijuana that gets you "high".

People grow hemp plants for their seeds and stalk. It's used for tex tiles, clothes, food, and other industrial purposes. A plant mus contain less than .3% of THC to be considered hemp.

Self-Care when you're feeling under the weather

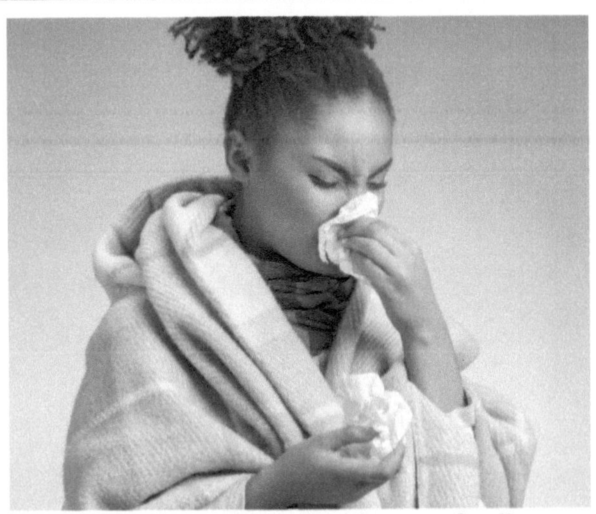

General dietary guidelines when you're not feeling your best whether it is from a head cold, flu, stomach upset, nausea, vomiting, constipation, diarrhea, or when recuperating from injuries, surgeries, or other illness.

-During convalescence & severe deficiencies: Eat cereal creams, rice congees, clear broth such as chicken or vegetable, light soups.

-Foods & Drink to Minimize: Raw cold foods, raw salads, ice cream, popsicles, frozen desserts, mangoes, watermelon, pears, celery, persimmons, cucumbers, iced-cold drinks, milk, cheese, commercial sweetened yogurts, sugar, white flour, tofu.

Gui Zhi Tang (Cinnamon Twig) mentioned previously in the section, FOOD AND THERAPY FOR IMPROVED BLOOD FLOW AND ANALGESIA is beneficial for the immune system and relieves symptoms of the common cold.

References

Duhigg, C. (2012). The Power of Habit: Why We Do What We Do In life And Business. New York: Random House Publishing Group.

Flaws, B. & Sionneau P. (2002). The Treatment of Modern Western Diseases with Chinese Medicine: A Textbook And Clinical Manual, New Expanded Edition. Boulder: Blue Poppy Press, Second Edition.

Flaws, B. (2008, Aug.). The Tao of Healthy Eating, Dietary Wisdom According to Chinese Medicine, Second Edition. Boulder: Blue Poppy Press.

Flaws, B. (1999). Welcome to There's a Fungus Among Us: A Talk on Chinese Medicine & Chronic Candidiasis. Lecture and Notes.

Gao, F., Li, M., Liu, Y., Gao, C., Wen, S., & Tang, L. Intestinal dysbacteriosis induces changes of T lymphocyte subpopulations in Peyer's patches of mice and orients the immune response towards humoral immunity. (2012, December 11). Retrieved from http://gutpathogens.biomedcentral.com/articles/10.1186/1757-4749-4-19

Graf, J, MD, & Bowman, A. (2008, December 30). Stop Aging, Start Living. The Revolutionary 2-Week pH Diet That Erases Wrinkles, Beautifies Skin, and Makes You Feel Fantastic. New York: Three Rivers Press.

Glover, S. and Girion, L. (2013, March 29). Prescription drug-related deaths continue to rise in U.S. *Los Angeles Times.* Retrieved from http://articles.latimes.com/2013/mar/29/local/la-me-ln-prescription-drugrelated-deaths-continue-to-rise-20130329.

Green, M. & Keville, K. (2012, July 25). Aromatherapy: A Complete Guide to the Healing Art. Crossing Press.

Gumenick, N. (2005). Classical Five-Element Acupuncture Program. Personal collection of N.Gumenick, The Institute of Classical Five-Element Acupuncture Inc., Santa Monica, CA.

Hadazy, A. (2010). Think Twice: How the Gut's "Second Brain" Influences Mood and Well-Being. Scientific American. Retrieved from https://www.scientificamerican.com/article/gut-second-brain/

Hosker, H. (2005). With over 200 hormones in the body doing hundreds of different jobs, it's important to keep them in balance. Joyce Walter looks at what you can do to maintain healthy levels. Institute for Optimum Nutrition. Retrieved from http://www.ion.ac.uk/information/onarchives/hormonesbalance

Johnson & Johnson. Prevention and Wellness. Retrieved from
https://www.jnj.com/sites/default/files/pdf/prevention-and-wellness.pdf

Johnson, R.K., Appel, L.J., Brands, M., Howard, B., Lefevre, M., Lustig, R., Sacks F., Steffen, L., Wylie-Rosett, J. (2009, Sept. 15). American Heart Association. Dietary Sugars Intake and Cardiovascular Health: A Scientific Statement From the American Heart Association. Retrieved from:
http://circ.ahajournals.org/content/120/11/1011.full.pdf

Johnson, S. (2015, July 14). Evidence-Based Essential Oil Therapy, The Ultimate Guide To The Therapeutic and Clinical Application of Essential Oils. Orem: Scott A. Johnson Professional Writing Services, LLC.

Johnson, S. & Plant, J. (2015, October 12). Synergy, It's An Essential Oil Thing. Orem: Scott A. Johnson Professional Writing Services, LLC.

Keown, D., M.B., Ch.B., L.Ac. (2014). The Spark in the Machine: How the Science of Acupuncture Explains the Mysteries of Western Medicine. London & Philadelphia: Singing Dragon.

Lesser LI, Mazza MC, Lucan SC. (May 2015). Nutrition Myths and Healthy Dietary Advice in Clinical Practice. Am Fam Physician. 2015

May 1;91(9):634638 retrieved from: ttp://www.aafp.org/afp/2015/0501/p634.html

u, H.C. (1999, April 01). Chinese Natural Cures: Traditional Methods for Remedies and Prevention. New York: Black Dog & Leventhal

Magrone, T. & Jirillo, E. (2013, August 05). The interplay between the gut immune system and microbiota in health and disease: nutraceutical intervention for restoring intestinal homeostasis. Affiliation: Department of Basic Medical Sciences, Neuroscience and Sensory Organs, University of Bari, Bari, Italy, Policlinico, P.zza G. Cesare 11, 70124, Bari, Italy. *Current Pharmaceutical Design*, 19(7): 1329-1342.

Monastyrsky, K. (2008, Oct. 15). Fiber Menace: The Truth About the Leading Role of Fiber in Diet Failure, Constipation, Hemorrhoids, Irritable Bowel Syndrome, Ulcerative Colitis, Crohn's Disease, and Colon Cancer. Ageless Press; 2nd edition.

Office of Disease Prevention and Health Promotion. (2015). Scientific Report of the 2015 Dietary Guidelines Advisory Committee. Part D. Chapter 1: Food and Nutrient Intakes, and Health: Current Status and Trends. Retrieved From: https://health.gov/dietaryguidelines/2015-scientific-report/06-chapter-1/d1-2.asp

Oviedo-Rondón, E.O., DVM, MSc., PhD., Dipl. ACPV. Dysbacteriosis, its causes and its impact. Prestage Department of Poultry Science, College of Agriculture and Life Sciences. North Carolina State University, Raleigh, NC 27695-7608. Retrieved from http://www.dsm.com/content/dam/dsm/anh/en US/documents/Dysbacteriosis,%20its%20causes%20and%20its%20impact.pdf

Pitchford, P. (1993). Healing with Whole Foods: Asian Traditions and Modern Nutrition. Berkeley: North Atlantic Books.

Prout, L. M.S. (2000, October 13). Live in The Balance: The Ground-Breaking East-West Nutrition Program. New York: Marlowe & Company.

Vane, JR, Botting, RM. (2003, June 15). The Mechanism of action of aspirin. Thromb Res. 110(5-6):255-8. From https://www.ncbi.nlm.nih.gov/pubmed/14592543/

Wilson, Lawrence. (2015, April). Your Intestinal Flora. Retrieved from http://drlwilson.com/ARTICLES/FLORA.htm

Worwood, V.A. (1991). The Complete Book of Essential Oils & Aromatherapy. Novato: New World Library.

About the Author

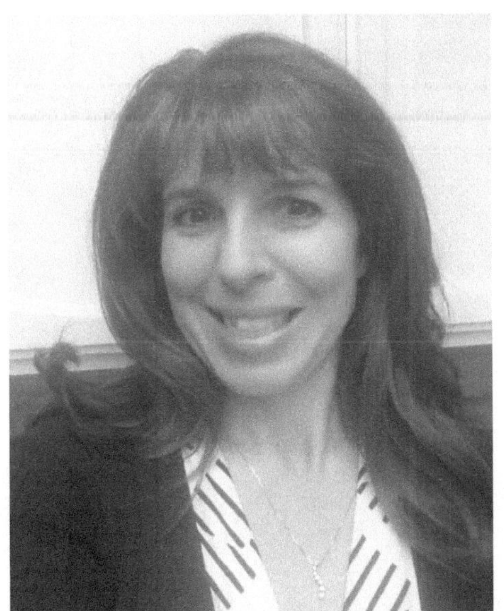

Dr. Michele Arnold has been practicing the healing art of Chinese Medicine and Acupuncture for over eighteen years. She is excited to share her experiences and expertise with you.

"It is my personal mission to spread the potential health benefits of nature's plant medicines. Herbs, spices, and essential oils can be used to cultivate a wellness lifestyle to enjoy a healthier, happier life-longer! Reach Your True-Potential, Naturally!